ESSENTIALISTISM: MASTERING THE ART OF LESS

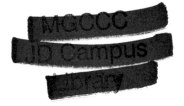

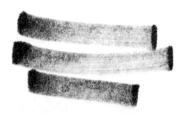

Table of Contents

INTRODUCTION

Greg McKeown was just another business executive who was constantly busy and on the move trying to do more things than he could. Like most other people, his response to any challenge was "work harder". That was until he discovered the "essentialist" movement. That was until he came to classify everybody as either being an essentialist or a non-essentialist. Buoyed by its teachings, Greg is now a frontline champion, devoted defender and material evidence of the benefits of minimalism. But how exactly did he make this transformation? How did he move from a busy executive trying to cram and stuff more items onto his do-to list to a perpetually free one?

Well, according to Greg in his widely-read book "Essentialism; the art of less", essentialism dwells on the concept of being available to do more by carefully picking the battles you fight. Half of the people on earth are constantly busy. The other half? Even busier!!! We get our energies and creative talents exhausted and weakened by constantly keeping them in action for unnecessary causes. We dilute our ability to make a positive change and reduce our odds of achieving more success by constantly applying them on the most mundane of matters; important and unimportant. The end result is that most people exhaust these abilities faster than they realize. Before they can scream Jack, they are already tired of doing everything without achieving much. How then can you make the same journey Greg made?

In the first place, it takes a trigger to actually convince people to embrace the notion that more is actually less. In Greg's case, it came with the delivery of his child. While his wife was in labor in the process of giving birth, he received a call that asked him to meet a prospective client to drop a pitch. What did yours truly do? Was he irrational enough to drop the pressing engagement he had at hand for the meeting? Could he be so blind enough to add further work pressure on top of the emotional and psychological ones he was having? Did he, like responsibility dictated, ignore the call and focus on the critical junction of his life unfolding right in his presence?

Of course he did not. Just like you and almost every other person on this planet would have, he couldn't ignore the chance to "do more". He added further trouble and upheavals onto the already existing ones. Like almost every other person, he ramped up the pressure on his brain and faculties of execution. He ran his mental ability and resilience into the ground. At the meeting, he couldn't focus on what was being discussed either. Yet, his mind also kept nagging at him. By piling up more pressure than he could handle, he achieved even further less than was expected. He lost the client and gained a sense of severe guilt at having left his life for the relatively nonessential act of meeting a new client. He neglected the important for the unnecessary. Do not get me wrong; a job interview is always important but in this case where he could simply have delegated or found some other ways of managing the situation such as postponement, he still found the verve and strength to take on more at the detriment of his already depleted mental reserve.

Before you throw stones though, look at yourself. What do you see? What life choices do you constantly take? Are you forever working and trying harder to achieve more? Have you left some vital things out for the less vital but more alluring options that promise instant gratification?

Now, take a step further; look at the people around you whom you come in contact with. Do you see more and more people who are seemingly always busy with one thing or the other; work, family, health etc? In fact, if you were critical enough, chances are you would realize you are one of them too. This is the era of being busy, where society has taught each and everybody to do as much as he can do; and then, some more.

It is not hard to see where the society picks this idea from though. The slogan "work harder" has forever been the bane of human endeavors. Under the illusion of achieving more through an exponential increase once effort is increased, more people have clogged up their schedules with vital and non-vital tasks. Nobody wants to be found lagging, so, most people create the illusion of being busy. They make up and create more action for themselves to be busy with. In truth though, they only end up creating more noise. They only end up choking up the already filled-up space that is their mind. The end result is that they end up like every other person; busy without too many results or proof of increased performance.

This is exactly what essentialism seeks to eliminate; the idea that more effort equals more success. Are you constantly overworked? Or do you exert so much effort and still feel like you are getting less value for the effort you have put in? Maybe there is even a hint of being underpaid somewhere in there? Do you work till your socks drop off daily without ever feeling like the results are never commiserate with the level of hard work you have put in? Is some part of your life suffering because of the other? Are you constantly almost estranged from the people closest to you?

If you are suffering from any of these signs above, it may be time to redefine your life goals and the way you go about trying to achieve them. It is time for you to jump on the essentialism train and set sail to go further than you ever thought. It is time for you to be free!!! And this is exactly why I have written yet another book on essentialism to help more people realize that by concentrating their firepower, they have a greater chance of forcing the walls and barriers in front of them open. Instead of focusing on too many targets at once at the risk of diluting your firepower, it is time for you to learn when to try and when to stop, how to select your battles and focus on the most important tasks.

Essentialism is a guide to being able to get more by having and doing less. But it is not the easiest path to tread. It requires a certain degree of resilience and willpower to not only change your lifestyle around but also your mindset. Mind you, changing your lifestyle without transforming your mindset is futile. Trying to do more without understanding or really subscribing to the ideas that essentialism preaches is a further waste of your time. You will eventually lapse into the hole you just tried to escape from. This is why it is important that you read this book with enough focus and concentration to enable you make that mindset change.

Do not get buoyed by the seemingly radical proposition that essentialism seems to represent to most people though. It takes only a single change in your mindset to change your perspective. You only need to be able to understand that you do not need to fill up every space in your day, schedule and mind with some task or the other just to feel like it is full and productive. In truth, the most creative and innovative personalities the world has ever seen regularly sought to free up enough space for their minds to grow and thrive. The Steve Jobs, Einsteins and Gates of this world did not need to take on more than they could handle. They simply focused on the most essential things they needed to succeed.

You can join them too on the trail to trailblazing success. Nothing is stopping you except for the fact that your mind is weighed down. This is the book to free your mind from all that weight. It is the defining blueprint for complete mental freedom and liberty to choose your own battles. Have a seat as I help you make a case for a better life.

PART ONE: DEMYSTIFYING ESSENTIALISM

"Essentialism isn't denial or self-scrutiny; it is a complete lifestyle that ensures that you are firing at the right targets rather than spraying your efforts around indiscriminately"

Essentialism means that you don't need to work hard or work at all to achieve success. In fact, the essentialist mind dictates that you should do less just for the sake of doing so. Essentialism dictates that you should wait interminably for the chance to act while keeping yourself busy with the luxuries and comfort of life.

Of course, the above description is a big, fat joke but nonetheless, it is what some people think of essentialism. Explain to the man out there on the streets that he should try to do less as a means to keeping his powder dry for the right occasion and he would instantly think you as being lazy or a chief procrastinator. This is why I will like to start the entire book with a part that seeks to clear out the misconceptions people have about essentialism.

Yes, essentialism says you should do lesser than you are doing currently. This may sound eerily similar to the tenets of procrastination and laziness but there is no further distance like the one between these two concepts and the rational life choice that is essentialism. Essentialism represents a conscious decision to remain in total control of how to act and when to act. It doesn't say; "STOP ACTING". It says "ACT WELL: ACT SMART". One of the greatest challenges people face while trying to understand and potentially embrace essentialism is that they fail to realize that most of what society and conventional wisdom dictates is not totally or factually true. Do not allow yourself get weighted down by some of these parochial views. Without further do, let us attempt to demystify and understand essentialism better in relation to its role as a life choice.

The essentialist versus the non-essentialist

Who is an essentialist? Or more appropriately, what does he seek to achieve? In what ways does he differ from every other person on the planet? First of all, let me borrow one of the concepts introduced by Mckeown. There are only two categories of people on Planet Earth; the essentialist and the non-essentialist. There is absolutely no grey areas or people who fall in between. You either decide to prioritize your actions consciously or you fall victim to the hustle and bustle that is most people lives.

Like you must have discerned, the most important difference between the essentialist and non-essentialist is their mindsets. While the non-essentialists tries to do so many things (most non-vital) at once, the essentialists understands that this is not compulsory. There is absolutely no reason or logic to expending all your efforts at once in various direction. Instead, he gathers his efforts and strength in a thundering ball of unstoppable energy and resilience that rolls surely and firmly in only a fewer directions at once.

With his efforts thus concentrated, it is no surprise that an essentialist is able to focus and ultimately win more battles than the non-essentialist. While essentialism is by no means the only ingredient for success, it can at the very least ensure that your greatest strengths are directed towards the most pivotal of your needs. In the first instance, essentialism enables you to sort out your needs and wants into two neat and clearly distinct piles. This means you are forever under no illusion as to what your next step or challenge should be.

In essence, the essentialist tries to achieve more by focusing his greatest strengths and advantages on a few, selected priorities while the non-essentialists runs around a bit aimlessly trying to kill two, four or ten birds with only one stone. This is the greatest difference between essentialists and non-essentialists.

The era of confusion

"The only judgment that you can make upon the world is that it is
confused"
-Marshall Vian Summers

The world today is a conflicting melting point of different ideas, opinions and thoughts. For the first time in human history, technology means that distances grow ever shorter and what used to be limits are getting erased faster than ever. Two, three centuries ago, the only way to get to know the minds of people far away from you was to listen to third-party reports and probably books but with the development of the internet and mass media, it means your ears are literally with every other person on the planet.

Thoughts and opinions fly at us at an increasingly alarming rate but it doesn't seem to matter to most people that our capacity to filter them out has not really been upgraded. Therefore, more and more people are living their lives according to what current societal norms, opinions, the media and most people say is right. Norms are very important but what happens when the trending train of thought around us is actually wrong or not factual enough; confusion. And that is exactly what the average man faces nowadays.

We receive so many ideas and opinions about what we should actually be doing or ascribing to be that we eventually, literally undergo a mental shutdown that means we put in a lethargic effort at almost everything. For most people now, they need new challenges and take on more tasks to prove that they are in line with the society's definition of hardwork as being busy. In the world today, the general opinion is that to be successful, you have to be busy; to be truly fulfilled and happy, you need to be there for everybody and be willing to contribute more than the limits of capacity. This means you may fall into the trap of thinking you need to appear busy at the very least to cultivate a social standing.

From this idea stems the harder, mental trap that says; do more. It is this idea that tells you to work harder today to make hay while the sun shines. Yes, it is necessary for you to put in enough work to guarantee or even give you a whiff at succeeding but the problem is that most people direct almost all of these efforts at so many things at once that the eventual reach and impact per each pursuit is much smaller compared to the exertions they have made? Why is this so? We discuss in the next chapter.

The "you can have it all" syndrome

We do not suddenly wake up one day and decide that we want to achieve so many things all at once. No!!! Society and its trappings do. Society dictates that we try to satisfy so many needs and wants, physical, financial and material, that we end up getting crushed under the weight of our expectations and the exertions we make to satisfy them. We want to be rich, have a fulfilled life, be healthy, socially respected and a thousand other things. Yes, we can be all of this but the problem lies in the fact that we want to be them in various dimensions.

As children, we are not sent to school any longer to get educated. Yes, it still remains the primary aim of going to school but education is no longer an end to itself. Rather, it is now a means for us to acquire the tools that will enable us be on the constant lookout for more and more opportunities. As such, from the day we can hold an opinion; we are constantly thought and programmed to look out for new opportunities to make more money, create value, be of help and service, be happy or share with others. These are all great ends on their own but when thrown into the proper context; the chase after all of them at once actually blunts our edge and our ability to react to changing needs.

From childhood, we no longer think we have choices on what we want to do. We constantly think we can have it all at the same time all at once. News flash; you cannot eat your cake and still have it. You cannot work yourself dog-tired for long hours every day and expect to feel fresh every other morning. You cannot to say yes to everything thrown at you and expect not to expend all the vital and useful reserve energy you kept for your own needs. One has to give for the other. It is either you satisfy most of your needs and some of your wants or try to mix them all together and hope to satisfy some from both ends. But experience dictates that you are likely to achieve fewer things from both categories.

The craze and craving to own and do everything and experience all the entire range of positive emotions is the greatest challenge you need to conquer to become essentialist in nature. Conquer it you must!!!

The novelty syndrome

This is the other side of the coin in relation to the "have-it-all" syndrome. This is an applied derivation of the syndrome in fact. Not every new thing is meant to be tried but sadly, few people realize this. That you have not done something before does not mean that you need to jump at the first chance to try it out. No!!! There must have been a reason why you hadn't taken the chance to perform those actions before.

It explains why the vast majority are constantly in need of more money and gratification. They feel they need new resources to acquire their attest and newest wants. The newest Android device, iPhone or an upgrade to their current vehicle; name it. We have been taught to want new possessions and strive to get them.

It is not just material items though. Society also dictates that we make new friendships always, try to break new ground regardless of whether it is actually favorable or not, find new ways to make ourselves indispensable and create new channels for more comfort and luxury. The end result; more tasks and things going on. These combine to form a large burden that most people cannot carry alone and eventually, there is a breakdown in mental capacity to achieve.

Quoting from my last book; "We become victims of the novelty craze. The novelty craze is inbuilt in us. It is what pushes us to get a larger house than we need; it is what keeps extra cars in our garage. It is why you can't say no to any request. It is why your life appears cluttered and crowded. The world today is filled with noise and too much static. Essentialism allows you to chart a path through all the noise so you can hear yourself." This is the essence of essentialism.

Redefining happiness and success

We all want to be happy and successful. There is no harm or wrong in this. Or is there? Improbable as it may seem and despite the fact that happiness and success are rightly the next most important thing we can ascribe to after survival, more people have hurt themselves and their psyches chasing happiness and success than in any other endeavor. This should makes you pause for a minute and wonder if happiness is worth chasing? Or more accurately, are we chasing the right sort of happiness, in the right way, for the right reasons and at the right cost? Consider the average Tom on the street and the chances are very high indeed that the answers to all the four questions will be negative. Why then do we still persist in overloading ourselves for the wrong causes? Let us attempt to redefine what happiness and success should look like as a first step to getting out of the clutches of the unnecessary burdens we place upon ourselves.

Do not get deceived; material possessions and wealth do not equal contentment. There are far more uncontented individuals among the wealthy than the poor. Money cannot buy happiness. It may purchase you some cheap illusion of happiness but as with all illusions, it will eventually fade. Defining your happiness by the society's standard of having enough to spend and even extra will lead you into a vicious cycle. You will forever try to reach certain milestones of wealth as a marker of happiness. But the sad reality is this type of thinking will forever shift your goalposts. For every milestone you reach, you will find the bar set just a bit above your head. So, you will need to work just a bit harder to get to the next milestone only to find the bar a bit above you again. You may enjoy this happiness but only for a little bit before you crave more. Most people overwork themselves chasing after these milestones that eventually count for naught.

Do not get me wrong; essentialism doesn't preach austerity or poverty. By all means, try to get reach; it is a great feeling to be wealthy. In contrast, essentialism says, prune out the excess to achieve the needful. Happiness and success is also dependent on contentment though. Try every possible best to maintain a sane balance between work, family, finances and health. Too much focus on any of these at the detriment of others will leave you needing to do too much to achieve success and happiness.

The power of choice/the power to choose

Peter Drucker sums up what the world and the average man thinks. He said; "In a few hundred years, when the history of our time will be written from a long-term perspective, it is likely that the most important event historians will see is not technology, not the Internet, not e-commerce. It is an unprecedented change in the human condition. For the first time—literally—substantial and rapidly growing numbers of people have choices. For the first time, they will have to manage themselves. And society is totally unprepared for it."

There are so many life choices to make now. We have literally an inexhaustible supply line of choices and options we can take. This state of affairs though can be quite overwhelming. In fact, to most people, it is overwhelming and this is why they end up getting a confused. Their confusion about what choices then leave them at a loss at what to do. They end up doing one of two things; choosing to do all or not making a choice at all. Both scenarios end up giving them too much to do.

Most people simply decide to try out every option and go down every path. Therefore, they combine a lot of different tasks and aims and become constantly busy. They no longer seek to distinguish between which is important and not. They simply make themselves available for any and everything. What do you think this decision results in? Of course, it is stress and a fine stretching-out of the resources they possess. They don't make choices; so, they believe inherently that every task and challenge is theirs to complete.

The other category of people does not bother to do all. They simply decide not to pick a choice or option and await the vagaries and winds of life and society to point out a direction for them. This means they react rather than act on their own intuition or in their own interests. It is therefore not surprising that when things get a bit tempestuous, they have nothing to buffet themselves against the bad conditions. They therefore get swept away too trying to either satisfy the society or save themselves.

In either case, the ignorance or inability to exercise choices leaves men incapable of taking the right path. Instead, they just overload and burden themselves with unnecessary tasks that dilute their strengths. This is why it is important for you to embrace essentialism. Essentialism is to be able to empower yourself with the choice to make choices. Essentialism teaches you to identify your needs, draw up a plan, prioritize the right actions, cut off unnecessary tasks and focus on the essentials that can bring you success fast without extra baggage or side effects.

Why Become an Essentialist

Having made a general case for why you should not just allow essentialism pass your mind in thinking, let us narrow down the specifics of why you should actually become a core essentialist.

- More Time. Essentialism gives you more control over your schedule. It allows you a means to create time for leisure and adequate rest. With essentialism, you cut out the extraneous activities that eat up your time. A lot of people cannot get some quality time alone to themselves because of the high number of commitments they have made. They fail to prioritize their needs and wants and allow their urges and desires to take over control of their day-to-day routine. Essentialism minimizes all these by drastically reducing the number of activities and tasks you take on daily, creating more time for you to employ in more creative endeavors.

- More quality and efficiency. This is the entire essence of the "less is more" essentialist slogan. Instead of focusing and dissipating your energy, skills and talent on so many tasks at once that you become exhausted and unable to give your best to all of them, you can now choose tasks wisely depending on the attributes you possess. This will ensure that you consistently produce more quality than quantity. It will mean that you consistently begin to produce better results with less effort. You can easily gain more efficiency by limiting the number of distracting or conflicting engagements you possess.

- Sharpen your focus. It is easy to get lost in the complex maze that society deigns to call hardwork. It is highly likely that you may get trapped in a whirlpool of constant action and activity without too much mobility to show. Having other tasks to think of and work towards can easily leave you bereft of focus on your primary goals. Eliminate the extra tasks and you will suddenly find life easier with more focusing ability available for you to tap into.

- Less mental burden. With the current state of society, it should be no great surprise to see that has been an upward surge in the number and severity of mental disorders in the world today. Statistics show that more people than ever before in history have problems bordering on stress, anxiety and depression. Do not get it twisted. Society's expectation is what triggers half of stress. We constantly overwork ourselves to make more money, occupy more spheres and funnily enough stay busy. These same expectations also turn some unfortunate individuals into a ball of nerves. Believing it is blow or bust, they work themselves up into pitiable mental conditions. The same thing goes for chronically depressed people. It is quite common to find a larger percentage of depressed people among those that society supposedly holds up for our admiration. The famous pop star, athlete or tycoon who has millions in his account isn't necessarily happy as a non-essentialists. He probably works harder each day to maintain or grow his profile or wealth with the end result that often, they become depressed with their lack of progress and boring routines. Break this loop by embracing essentialism and laser-tailoring your effort towards the most important needs. This will help you feel free of the literal mental burden that most people carry along with them.

- Better health. Essentialism is a lifestyle not just an act. It covers virtually every aspect of life including your nutrition and health. By freeing up more time, you can plan to add regular exercise to your daily schedule. A vast majority of those who do not exercise regularly put it down to a lack of time to spare. In comes essentialism to open up the door for exercise to come in and improve your state of health. Also, with less mental burdens and more rest, you can finally start to plan how to get onto the next level of the health spectrum.

- More meaningful relationships. Divorce rates have never been this high before. While a number of reasons have contributed to this spike in separation and breakdown of relations, a lack of attention and time has always been a leading factor. Do you also constantly work yourself dog-tired during the day and consequently return home tired and grumpy? Well, many people do and this does not help them in any way protect their relationships. It isn't just marriages either that need more attention. All your relationships would be better if you could just prune out some of the activities and tasks that take up all of your time and attention, and start to show some attention to the people around you now.

- Developing contentment. Fulfillment and contentment are the real measures of happiness. They are the right ingredients that can ensure that you can escape the clutches of the "novelty craze". Therefore, essentialism is a key ally in the battle to get contented and satisfied with what you have, even if you must aspire for more.

PART TWO: THE ESSENTIALIST MINDSET

"Only once you give yourself permission to stop trying to do it all, to stop saying yes to everyone, can you make your highest contribution towards the things that really matter."
-Greg Mckeown

A great difference exists between the essentialist and the non-essentialist: they are two opposites and for that reason, shifting from one to the other, changing from being a non-essentialist to being an essentialist requires the right mindset. It is to help the reader adopt the right mindset that this part has been carefully written. The right mindset, the mindset of an essentialist, is one you must adopt and cultivate throughout your life. Nothing great has ever been achieved without enthusiasm. By enthusiasm here, I mean motivation coupled with dedication and the right efforts; enthusiasm in our own context is the right mindset which must persist right from now, when you are just coming into essentialism, to the end of your life.

That is because it is your mindset that will not only help you take the first essentialist step, but also ensure that you keep firm on the essentialist path. It will help you find the journey or lifestyle easy so that when in the process of cutting out the unimportant excess in your life you get stuck, you can easily dredge up the resilience module from your neural programming in the same way computer programs call up troubleshooting functions when they encounter problems performing the tasks they are designed to perform. You no doubt now know the essentialist mindset is nothing but conditioning your mind for the lifestyle. After all, is it not true that we are made of basically two things: our thoughts and actions? I shall now turn to discussing the important points in the essentialist mindset.

Willpower

Like every other endeavor or undertaking, essentialism, too, requires willpower in its adoption. What do I mean by this? Imagine wanting to quit smoking; imagine having the desire to do just that, to quit smoking, but lacking the willpower to do so. Your wishes would be as good as trying to make horses in a picture gallop. In simple terms, wishes are different from willpower. Wishes remain wishes until you fuel them with the right sort of mindset and willpower. While our wishes are mere desires, willpower identifies the state of mind that is set or ready to take on things, to get things done. It is willpower that gets you up from the bed in the morning and puts you in front of a desk to write out an application for the job. It is willpower that keeps you going even when you are slightly confused, hesitant or reluctant to take action. How does the willpower work then? Two ways: "a definite resolve to do" and "a continuous conviction" about the resolution. How do these two work together in synergy to help you bring out the best in you?

You need first of all to decide, firmly and clearly in your mind, that you want to adopt the essentialist lifestyle. The effect of this, after you make that decision, should be as if you have just sent a resignation letter to your boss. How does it feel when you do that? Permanent, right? Your resolution to do must be carefully thought out but you arrive at it. How do you do this? First, read this book to the end; this will help you carefully think about your decision or resolution so that when you finally resolve, it will not be as though you had only arrived at the decision by just a whiff of thought.

After that, what comes next is continuous conviction about the rightness of your resolution. How do you achieve this second leg of adopting the right mindset? Remember, first, that the mindset runs from the beginning of your journey to the end. So, at every stage in your journey when it seems to you that you have made the wrong decision, all you need do is remind yourself of the cluttered life you lived as a non-essentialist.

In other words, you need to remind yourself of the advantages of essentialism and how it can help you get the most out of your life. If you have already begun the essentialist journey, then all you need to do is to remind yourself of the many wins you have had so far since you decided to lead the essentialist lifestyle.

Positivity

Did you know your mind influence the results of your action in ways unimaginable? YES, our mind is the vehicle for all actions, conscious and subconscious. It directs our every step without us even noticing its role. It is because of this simple fact that you need to be positive about your ability to adopt the essentialist lifestyle and gain the essentialist gain or achieve the end goals. You need to adopt a positive attitude towards it.

I am not saying it is a very easy thing to do; imagine having to decide you need to let go of an undertaking you care so much about but which is achieving no good results to warrant you continuous attention. Making such a decision is one thing you will learn to do as an essentialist. I know this because I have myself been there. And that is why I am counseling positivity as one of the foundations upon which your life as an essentialist should be laid.

Positive thinking about your ability to get there, to achieve the goal, to become an essentialist is important because with its opposite, with negative thinking or negativity, you will end up setting yourself up as obstacle against your own achieving the goal. A mind that keeps telling itself of its own limitation is only working its own failure. Negative thinking is like trying to break free from slavery while at the same time forging the metal that is the bars of your prison. It is as erecting invisible roadblocks for yourself so that each time you decide to race; you keep crashing into these obstacles without knowing they are even there. It is therefore important to adopt a positive attitude towards your ability to becoming an essentialist. You need to adopt a "Yes-I-Can" attitude now and always or else you will never take the first step in this journey of freedom though you will think you have. Remember, if others have done it, you, too, can.

Why you should miss out

Our society is designed to make us feel we need more and have to be more and should be doing more. But like I stressed earlier, this is not always true or the prudent course of action. We have been wired to think that failing to pick up the freebies from the stores we buy from, is missing out on a great opportunity. But that it is free does not mean you should have it. What determines whether you should have it is if you need it I the first place; it is whether without it, life would be difficult. And it is often rare to find the very items we need being given out at no cost in stores. The same logic applies to those instances where we find items on discounts in stores. But beyond mere missing out on items, there is missing out on what seem to be real opportunities.

Get one thing straight: as an essentialist, what you are missing out on is not something you should seek in the first place. It is usually the things that come to you without you making efforts for it, something which seeks you rather than you seeking it out. Imagine being asked to take on a project which seems promising while you already are executing one. You did not seek out the second and you are already doing something important, executing a project you have carefully chosen out of possible many.

Let us consider another illustration before I analyze the two in terms of missing out. You really want to study computer engineering and you are already doing that in a respectable college. Then you got a fully-paid scholarship to study abroad in a better college, but the program now is not computer engineering; it is economics. The university is much more prestigious than the one you currently attend. You think what an opportunity! You could do well studying economics and possibly get a scholarship for your postgraduate studies. But if you reject economics, you are missing out on scholarships. How do you deal with this?

While it may seem you are wasting a great opportunity, focus instead on what you are already doing. Focus on how much your present undertaking means to you. Computer engineering is your passion, your dream and your aspiration. You even have a knack for it. It comes so easy to you. And truly, you could excel at economics and it is free. But it will not give you fulfillment or joy. One extra project means one more commitment; one more set of worries and possibly, one more great loss. Missing out now means you are focusing on maximizing your efforts on your present engagement

Now matters most

Now matters and now first! What do I mean by this? I am not advocating for a nonchalant attitude to the past or the future. But one thing must be clear: the past is gone and the future is yet to come. What matters is to live in the present, the moment, to the fullest while at the same time making the right decisions capable of allowing your future choices and undertakings key into the timelines in our lives like the edges of pieces in a puzzle. The past is certain because it has come and gone, and because we now have all the facts, we see better in retrospect. It should however not be allowed to haunt our present and our future. In the same vein, while it is normal to think and plan for the future, it is not healthy to worry sick about it – this will not remove the many uncertainties with which the future is always beset. What is important is to live the present moment right and ease gently into the future. Besides, does the future not start immediately after now?

So far, in this part, you have been provided with a glimpse into the essentialist mindset. It is a mind imbued with the willpower to do. It is not chained in negativity. It is a mind that focuses on the job of missing out rather than the fear of missing out. It knows that one's refusal to take on more means less worries and an opportunity to give one's best to the present one. In the part that follows, we shall start walking the essentialist way. I invite you to start the next chapter where we shall focus on prioritizing and cutting out the excess in our lives.

PART THREE: PRIORITIZING AND CUTTING OUT THE EXCESS

"Essentialism is not about how to get more things done; it's about how to get the right things done. It doesn't mean just doing less for the sake of less either. It is about making the wisest possible investment of your time and energy in order to operate at our highest point of contribution by doing only what is essential."
_ Greg Mckeown

What you have been doing so far in this book is like installing the operating system on your hardware. Our body is just like this: our mind and body are the hardware, and our mindset is the operating system which facilitates the use and activities of both the hardware and other application programs. You no doubt get the point here: the previous chapters have laid the foundation for the following chapters in this part of the book.

In this part, our focus will be on helping you start the very process of becoming an essentialist. You have taken the first step already. But in the parts that follow, you shall take further or more decisive steps in this river. You are only so far ankles deep in the water; you need to be submerged in it and that is exactly what the following chapters will try to help you achieve gradually.

Classifying Things and Actions: Important Vs Necessary Vs Unnecessary

This is the first thing you need to learn as an essentialist. You must learn and master the art of categorizing or classifying. The essence is that it helps you make definite sense of things. With categorizing, you can clearly demarcate things, people and activities in your life into different groups with different properties. It may sound strange that you really have to do this. It may also seem difficult to do. But by the time you finish doing it though, you will realize that it works.

The things you need to classify in your life are people, things and activities. You will notice virtually everything you do revolves around these. You relate with people in and outside of the home. You need them to do one thing or the other for you. Some depend on you to get things done and you, too, depend on others. People are the basis of your relationships; they define it. Without people, there would be no relationships.

Things in our context are materials. As humans, we cannot survive without one material possession or the other. Even the great ascetics had material possessions. Minimalist as Gandhi was, he still had a few items of possession until his death. Things get things done for us and they can represent memories and/or sentiments.

Activities are those things you engage in virtually all the time. Reading this book is an activity. Sitting and planning out your next project is an activity. Playing video games is an activity. Spending time at the bar with your friends or playing poker or merely sitting at the park in the evening are all activities. The list of what constitutes activity is endless.

The triad described above can all fall into three groups as to whether you need them or not. They could be: **primary**, **secondary** or **periphery**. They are primary if they are very important to you. In other words, a person, a thing or an activity can be of primary importance to you and by this we mean such person, thing or activity is indispensable. You cannot do without them. By now a number of things should have come to your mind. Your wife, children, parents and some of your closest friends fall into this category. They are the type of persons whom you can bleed for and go the extra mile for. The point being made is just that you can do anything for them because you can be sure they can do anything for you. They can hang themselves out to dry for you just as you can do the same for them. In terms of things, those material possessions of yours which you depend on for one reason or the other fall into this category, and so do those activities. Examples of these might be your clothes, car, laptop, phone, eating, bathing, studying, communicating etc.

The secondary group of persons, things or activities is those which are similar to those in the primary group but do not come close in comparison to the primary group. The reason is that while they are necessary for one reason or the other, they can be dispensed with. Think here of your boss, close friends, extended family members like your cousins etc. of things and activities, we might have here such examples as attending the book club meetings or meting of organizations, a bunch of your possessions which you still cling on to for sentimental purposes etc.

The periphery group identifies those persons, things and activities that are unnecessary but that you have in your life for one reason or the other. Your co-workers, a major bunch of your FB friends and interactions, members at your book club etc will fall into this category.

Do not get me wrong here. They all have roles they play. They are an integral and wanted part of your schedule but when they come with so much excess baggage that they threaten to affect or overwhelm your priorities, it may be time to get rid of them or at least minimize their impacts.

Set up a checklist and Shuffle

In the previous chapter, you learned how to classify people, things and activities in your life into categories depending on their importance to you. In this chapter, you will be taken through the process of identifying which one of these are your priorities. To do this, you need to use a checklist. The classification you have done in the previous chapter should here be reduced into writing and classified accordingly. Once you have done that, what comes next is prioritizing them and to do this, you may have to move these people, things and activities around. What should you consider moving?

Remember, the goal is to cut out the excess in your life, to help you become an essentialist and remain so. And as has been stated several times in this book, tough decisions have to be made, thanks to the nature of our society which has facilitated the cramping up of our lives with the non-essential things. To help you make that decision, consider the following about each of these groups: whether they positively, negatively or neutrally impact your life.

You are of course safe with the positive ones so you will retain them. And to determine whether they are positive, reflect on whether they aid or hinder your progress in life. Obviously, they should be aiding you in realizing your full potentials. They are negative if they hinder your progress in life. Remember, your progress in life includes your personal growth and development, physical, psychological or material. While some of these can be positive or negative, some may overlap the two and some others may be neutral. Those that overlap fall more on one side than the other side, and those that are neutral influence your life neither positively nor negatively.

While it is clear you are to retain the positive ones, what to do with the negative ones that fall in the primary or secondary group is to not cut them out immediately. Attempts must be made by you to change them into things that will positively impact your life. It is only upon failure on such attempts that you can begin to think of cutting them out. As to the negative ones in the periphery group, they need not be corrected. They are unnecessary in the first place. Cut them out once and for all.

The positive ones in the periphery groups, can, if possible, be migrated into the secondary group. But this should not be automatic; it is only what you should do when you realize you had wrongly classified it in the first place. That someone, something or an activity is beneficial to you does not necessarily mean you should keep it. If there are other important things that fulfill its goal in the first place, then you need not keep it. Remember, it is not necessary for you in the first place and that is why it is in the periphery group; and the goal of essentialism is to retain only the few that matter and work for you.

The "Definite Yes" test

At times we find it difficult to decide whether something is good or bad for us. We find it difficult to take on an endeavor, especially when you have become wary of taking on too many tasks than you need. If you have just taken on the essentialist mindset, you may at times find it difficult to determine whether to accept or retain something. This doubt no doubt sets in because that thing partially convinces us of its essence. Yet, such conviction might only be on the face of it. What should you do in such an instance?

Adopt the "Definite Yes" test. What do I mean by this? I am saying go for total conviction. Allow me to borrow a legal term to describe the type of conviction being described here. A person standing trial for an offence must be linked to the offence beyond reasonable doubt but not without the shadow of doubt. The courts will say his guilt need not be proven to the hilt. But, in our case, you need to subject the said decision to the extreme test of "to the hilt". It is either you are totally convinced of the need to take on the undertaking or you are not taking it up at al. That is, you need to set a conviction benchmark of 100% so that what you want to do, the person you want to hire, the investment you want to pursue, must be 100% before you take on the task, hire the person or pursue that investment.

If you allow a shortage of 20%, then you should not be surprised if in the long run the shortage increases in percentage. A simple illustration to get this point is when you are hiring someone to fill a vacancy in your organization, say the sales department, you should not bring onto the team someone who in the long run or even at the outset will need padding and patching. Why? He will slow you down and if care is not taken, they are likely to cost you a great deal.

The Polite "No" and Trade-offs

In this chapter, the focus is to help you master two interrelated arts: the art of the "Polite No" and the art of "Trade-offs". One thing essentialism wants to help you achieve is gaining more time, energy and resources for only the things that matter in your life. In the previous chapter, you learned about prioritizing and cutting off the excess and unnecessary things in your life. While the discussion here will be focused on something similar, it will be more tailored to how you will not get your life clogged again once you take the first step of cutting out the said excess.

One thing we often find difficult to do as humans is saying "No" to others. The reasons for not wanting to do this may vary from one person to another. In some instances, it could stem from your desire to be seen as the good Samaritan, the one who comes to the aid and rescue of every one in need. Your own reason may be different; perhaps you just do not want to be seen as a bad person. Or perhaps the person is all too important for you to say "No" to. It may even fall under the false notion that only you can fix their problem; this last reason is usually the one many people give themselves. But there is a big fallacy in it. It is in fact crystallized as a mental disorder; co-dependency.

The truth is that people really do not care who gets their problems fixed. All they really care about is that it gets fixed. By whom and how it was fixed, I repeat, does not really matter to them. So, the question you should ask yourself is whether it matters that you say "Yes" to them considering that they can get the problem fixed by some other persons or means and especially that you do not have the luxury of time to engage them or whatever it is they want you to do. Mind you, I am not asking you not to help others. I am only saying when you want to do so; it should not be at your utter inconvenience. Service to humanity is in fact giving up yourself for the service or to the aid of others. And as I state earlier in this book, people in your primary relationship group are the only ones you can really do so much for.

While contemplating what to do, whether to say "Yes" or "No", always remind yourself that if you say "Yes" to every request, you are allowing others to decide for you where to invest your time and energy. If you let this go on, you are soon to lose sight of your own focus – you will find your calendar filled with time you are giving to others with none left for yourself and the things you passionately care about or should care about or should in fact do. As Tim Ferris said; "What you don't do determines what you can do".

When people approach us safe in the knowledge that we cannot say "No" to their requests, there are two strategies we can employ: the "Delayed Yes" tactics and/or the "Polite No". Rather than saying "No" to them immediately, tell them you need more time to think about it or check some things out to be able to see if you can help. Then, later, send them a polite message or an email saying you regret that you could not help as your schedule is already filled up. Or you could say "No" immediately but only in a polite manner that tells them you have other important things to do. Consider saying something like: "Regrettably, I cannot help at the moment for this reason or another" or "I think I am not in the best position right now to help". The situation and the person should determine the manner in which you present your "No".

Must it be you? Delegating, Leveraging or Outsourcing

Yes, you might just be the one filling up your life with too many activities or tasks or projects than you should ordinarily take on or than you can even take on. The end result of this is not doing any of the tasks well. How do you avoid this? There are three ways I am suggesting: delegating, leveraging and outsourcing.

Perhaps you are a do-it-all person so that despite the fact that you have employees, colleagues, associates or friends who could do different things for you, people at your back and call, you still resort to doing things yourself. Nothing eats into your time faster than this. Learn to delegate; this will be easy to do if you have used the principle of the "Definite No" in employing people who work for you as you can be quite sure they will give you the best result for the job.

Leveraging is another thing you should do. It is the art of using other people's resources to get something done for yourself, albeit not dishonestly.

Delegating tasks to your employees can be a form of leveraging but what if you do not have employees? Must you do everything yourself? This is when we talk of leveraging on other people's time, money and skills. Why should you put all of your own money into an investment? Can you not get others to finance the business for you to get it up? The story is told of how Bill Gates' partner was going to withdraw his funding while Microsoft was still nothing and it is said that Bill Gates begged him not to withdraw his shares but instead count it as a loan. This simply shows the art of leveraging on other people's money. The moment you seek you cannot do something yourself, outsource it to someone who can. Thanks to technology, outsourcing jobs to freelancers has never been much easier.

Plugging the resources drain

If you still wonder how you lose a lot of money or time or energy or resources, then you should check yourself for sunk-cost bias which I have described in this chapter as resource drains. What do resource drains do or how do they work? It is simple: the effect that you have already invested so much in a failing project tricks you into investing more in it, in the hope that it just might work when in fact you are near certain that nothing good can come out of it. You then keep committing more time, money and resources because of this self-induced delusion. The effect is that you keep losing so much and you keep rationalizing it. And for as long as you keep up this charade or commitment, you will lose sight more and more of the reality of things until you are neck deep in the very things that add no value whatsoever to you.

Play and Rest

Indeed, many underestimate the importance of these two to our lives. And the truth is that without them, we would be like overworked horses. There must be time for work and so there must be for play and equally rest. What makes these two important? It is scientific fact beyond any possible rebuttal that the body needs to play and rest. And, before I go further, I should state that these two are not the same.

Play is the means by which we refresh our spirit during the day. It is a temporary fix for boredom and tiredness, especially while we are engaged at a task. Playing or having fun can equally give us inspiration about the things we do. Einstein often talks about how he daydreams about some of the things that later became his scientific theories.

Rest, on the other hand, can include play, too. But the rest I am talking about here is sleep. It has been scientific established that we need about eight hours of sleep in a day. It is during sleep that the brain catalogues all the information we have received during the day. It also helps the body refresh its systems and get us ready for the following day. If you think that for every minute we spend sleeping, there is a decrease in productivity, then you are caught in a web of fallacies. The appropriate measure of sleep does not decrease productivity. On the other hand, it increases creativity which leads to better ideas to gain on time and resources. You must structure your day and activities in such a way that they leave room for you to devote some time to rest and doing the things you derive joy from doing.

CONCLUSION

The word "priority" was introduced into the English dictionary in the fifteenth century. It was singular. It meant the most important aim and goal people had. It remained a word with no plural for the next five hundred years until we decided to dilute its potency by pluralizing it. And from that moment to today, the average number of priorities the average man gives himself to complete has continued to rise steadily. We have continued to find new pursuits to make even when our resources, physical, mental, emotional or financial, are stretched thin. We continuously try to seek an elusive true happiness and have had to settle for a watered-down version for so long as a society that our first goal now, is to be busy doing something or the other.

Has this brought us true happiness or success? Has dividing our abilities and efforts into small branches and offshoots helped us make a big, consistent impact? Has keeping yourself busy to the point of exhaustion helped you make giant strides? The secret to fast and consistent success is being able to conserve and concert our energy and efforts at our goals in small batches. When we do this, we can make one fell swoop for success rather than start trying to chip away the wall in front of us in different places all at once. This is the essentialist way and principle.

Know this one thing; for so long as you wish to be busy, for as long as you cannot bring yourself to be able to say "No" and reject offers that do not really add value, you will always find other people and activities ready to creep in and help you fill up the spaces and freedom in your life. You will always be busy at your own detriment. Essentialism asks that you prioritize and know what you have and need to do. Essentialism helps you define a straight path aimed at your goal and safeguards you against setting off along long-winded detours that waste your chances ad efforts.

Lin Yutang was absolutely right when he said; "the wisdom of life consists in the elimination of non-essentials". Pick your goals, set your priorities and allow this guide every conscious and subconscious action you take. Do not get deceived or brow-beaten into thinking you do not have a choice or say in what happens to you or your life. In fact, as Madeleine L'Engle aptly summarized; "It is the ability to choose that makes us human". When you do go to make your choices though, think only of the essentials; the things and people who are most vital to you in that moment. Do not hesitate to say

"No"; do not dither in delegating or leveraging other people's abilities. This is the way of the essentialist.

ACT LESS TO ACHIEVE MORE!!!

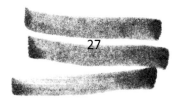

$13.37

3/20/18